Watchers

Freestyle 2019
Recipes with
Smartpoints
and Healthy
Diet Program

Dylan Cooper

Table of Contents

Weight Watchers as Freestyle

Every food and drink has a Smart Points value. one easy-to-use number that's based on calories, saturated fat, sugar, and protein. You are assigned a Smart Points budget that nudges you into making healthier eating choices, while staying satisfied and seeing weight-loss results. Zero Points foods category is made up of lean proteins, fruits, and vegetables. These foods provide a foundation from which you can build a healthy pattern of eating without imposing a great risk of overeating, so it's easier to pay attention to when you feel satisfied, rather than overeating them. For instance, it's much harder to eat six chicken breasts than six cookies. Weight watchers Freestyle will help you find an activity that fits your life. Doing what you enjoy instead of what you think you "should" do is the key to sticking with physical activity.

Finding success with weight loss is about being in the right frame of mind. With Weight watchers Freestyle, you'll learn new skills and techniques to help you shift your mindset. Because if you think differently you'll act differently. A shift in your mindset will help you gain greater self- awareness to make different choices, so you can achieve your goals and become a happier, healthier you. The Smart Points system has been incredibly successful in helping members to eat better while losing weight, but we are always looking to make the program even simpler and more enjoyable for you. Weight Watchers is designed to change your relationship with food. They do this with a point system that is cleverly designed to make less healthy choices "cost" more points. Smart Points are based on calories, saturated fat, sugar, and protein. If a food is high in saturated fat or sugar, it's going to cost you more points. If it's high in protein, it will have a lower point value, even if it has the same number of calories as another item.

For example, a typical store bought donut has about 208 calories, and nearly 9 grams of sugar. This donut is going to be 8 Smart Points. In contrast, 3 ½ ounces of lean rib eye roast has 216 calories, yet only 5 Smart Points. This is because the beef has no sugar, is high in protein, and only has 4.4 grams of saturated fat. If you're like me, eating the beef will keep you from being hungry for several hours. The donut will leave you peckish in about an hour. If the math in the above paragraph has your head exploding, don't worry about it. All the calculations are done for you. All you need to do is bring up your tracker (electronic) and punch in the food you ate. If you can't do it right at the moment you ate, take a quick picture with your smartphone and use the image to jog your memory later.

Zero Point Foods

Based on successful Smart Points system, Weight Watchers Freestyle offers more than 200 zero Points foods including eggs, skinless chicken breast, fish and seafood, corn, beans, peas, and so much more to multiply your meal and menu possibilities. And it makes life simpler too. You can forget about weighing, measuring, or tracking those zero Points foods. By combining zero Points foods and foods with Smart Points values, you have more freedom when building meals and snacks, along with the flexibility to have a satisfying meal no matter how the day or week went. Zero points foods are one of the things that people love the most about the Weight Watchers program but for some they can lead to slower weight loss if they are overused. This is especially true when it comes to lean proteins, beans and legumes, eggs, and fruit. It is important to have a full understanding about the zero points, your cravings to the kinds of food that provides the point, and how to stay consistent on the tolerable ones.

How it Works

While there is no totally free option for Weight Watchers directly, there are tons of options out there to keep you in your budget. First things first, Weight Watchers won't have a free option, but they do offer tons of deals around the holidays and the new year. To do this on your own, you'll have to do a lot of guesswork to figure out what your daily and weekly point values are going to become. The lowest points per day that the new option is giving is 23 Smart Points per day. The lowest weekly points would be 14 Smart Points per week. This will vary greatly depending on the person, their weight, goal weight, height, sex, and activity level. Tracking is still the backbone of the program. Recording (as accurately as possible) what you eat each day is the thing that keeps you accountable for your choices. And trust me; you have a lot of choices. Unlike other commercial programs that require you to eat "their" food (you all know which ones I'm talking about); on Weight Watchers you can literally eat anything you want. Just not all at once!

Another key point that remains the same is reframing how you think about food. Food is fuel for your body, not a "friend" to turn to when the going gets rough. Also there is a continued emphasis on moving your body more, and sitting less. Now that there are so many zero point foods, how are you supposed to takeoff weight? Well, that brings me to an important point. Just because you can eat all these zero points foods, doesn't mean you should stuff yourself on them. In fact, you should eat until you're satisfied, not until you can't put another bite in your mouth. This should seem like common sense, but needs to be remembered and reinforced. Also, with regard to food choice, you should try to vary your routine from time to time. For example, if you have a skinless chicken breast with lettuce for lunch every single day, you might lose weight. You might also lose the joy of eating! Being on Weight Watchers can be an epicurean adventure, limited only by your imagination. Pay attention to the flavors and textures of your food choices, and try new recipes. There are always new ideas online, as well as in the program literature. You are bound to find something that you like.

Weight Watchers have proven that the program has helped in achieving their dream shape and body size. Some of the experience that had been shared by participants includes:

- Participants said they had fewer food cravings and less hunger.
- Nearly three out of four were satisfied with their weight loss progress at six months.
- More than 93 percent agreed WW Freestyle helps them feel healthier.
- And of those who've tried to lose weight before, more than 82 percent agreed that WW Freestyle is easier to do and almost 93 percent agreed it gives them more flexibility in their food choices compared to other times they've tried to lose weight in the past.

Weight watchers food lists

One of the main features of the Weight Watchers program is their point system. All foods are given a points value and your goal on the program is to stay within your daily points allowance. However, anyone who has dieted before knows that when hunger strikes, it can be difficult to stay on track. That's why Weight Watchers offers a wide variety of healthy food options that have zero Smart Points. These zero Points foods can be eaten freely on the plan and are a great way to stay within your daily target. Under the newest Weight Watchers plans. There are a bunch of new zero point's foods! Hooray! The new list now includes lean proteins like eggs, chicken breast, and turkey. It also includes beans and legumes like chickpeas, black beans, and lentils as well as nonfat plain yogurt and tofu. This is in addition to the fruits and vegetables that were zero points in the previous plans. The Weight Watchers food list will make it much easier to create a lower point meal and since protein is now a part of the list, it will be easier to stay full with zero points options. The only concern is that it will be much easier to potentially overeat. The new zero points foods have more calories and if you are eating too many, it could be possible to gain weight on the new plan.

The new Flex and Freestyle plan now include lean animal and plant based protein sources like chicken, turkey, eggs, tofu, lentils, beans, and yogurt. Plus, you can now enjoy sweetcorn and peas for free on the new plans. Specifically, here are the new zero points foods for the new WW plans. Boneless skinless chicken breast

- Boneless skinless turkey breast Ground lean chicken
- Ground lean turkey
- Thin sliced deli chicken breast Thin sliced deli turkey breast

- All fish and shellfish (this does not include smoked or dried fish) Canned fish that is packed in water or brine (i.e. canned tuna or canned salmon in water) Tofu and smoked tofu
- Quorn fillets, ground Quorn, and Quorn pieces (meat substitute) Eggs
- Nonfat plain regular and Greek yogurt Plain soy yogurt

Fresh, frozen, and canned beans and lentils that are packed without oil or sugar (Lentils, chickpeas, black beans, pinto beans, kidney beans, split peas, soy beans, and more). Also, most vegetables are zero points on the new Flex and Freestyle plans. This means you can enjoy most non-starchy vegetables for zero points on the plan. Just be aware that you do need to count any oil or butter the vegetables are cooked with. There are a few vegetables that are not zero points including potatoes, sweet potatoes, yams, parsnips, cassava, mushy peas, yucca, and olives. This includes fresh, frozen, and canned vegetables as long as they aren't packed with any additional oil, sugars, or fats.

On the new Weight Watchers plans, almost all fruits are zero points but they should be eaten in moderation since they can quickly add up. The only exceptions to this are avocados and plantains. Also it is important to know that when you blend fruit in a smoothie, it is no longer counted as zero points. The reason for this is that a smoothie contains much more fruit than we would normally eat in one sitting. For example, someone would rarely sit down and eat a banana, a cup of berries, a mango, and some pineapple in one sitting but isn't rare to see this in a large smoothie. This includes fresh fruit as well as frozen, canned, or jarred fruit as long as it is packed without additional sugar. The last category of zero points food in the WW plans are for things like spices, low calorie and low sugar condiments, and many things we use to enhance the flavour in recipes. Some examples of these ingredients include things like vinegars, broth, fresh and dried spices and rubs, mustard, hot sauce, capers, and salsa. Please note, that some of these ingredients do have points depending on the amount you are using. They may be zero points for a small serving but if you are using more in a recipe, they may contain more points. There is no doubt that zero points foods are one of the things that people love the most about the Weight Watchers program but for some they can lead to slower weight loss if they are overused. This is especially true when it comes to lean proteins, beans and legumes, eggs, and fruit. Generally, you should try to eat zero points foods in moderation and only until you are full. Try not to overeat, watching portion sizes, even if it is zero- point food. For example, even though eggs are zero points with the new plan, it still isn't a good idea to have a 4 or 6 egg omelette for breakfast. Instead opt for a 2-3 egg omelette, which is closer to a standard portion size.

Additionally, if you find your weight loss is slowing or plateauing, it may be a good idea to look at how you are using zero point foods. Many people find that they may be over using these foods and when they cut back, their weight loss picks up again. Again, this is just a strategy to consider if your weight loss isn't progressing as you would like. If it is - then just keep doing what you are doing!

Let's count the fats you can lose

Weight Watchers works by assessing each member by age, weight, height and gender, then determining how much food he or she needs to eat to lose weight at what the company calls a safe rate one to two pounds per week. The member is assigned a daily point target, and spends those points on food. Some foods—fruit and vegetables especially—have zero points. Foods full of simple sugar and fat tend to have high points value. Where an apple is zero points, a slice of apple pie is 12 points. Members are encouraged to track everything they eat, which can be done offline, online, or via an app. Some members had proven to had lost 1-2lbs per week. Most weight watchers should except a range such as this during the program. The weight change also leads to a change in your points. Therefore, attention must be paid to the points and weight loss correlation. The lack of restrictions makes the plan easy to work. You can literally eat anything you want on Weight Watchers, so long as you account for it and structure the rest of your intake around it accordingly. Weight Watchers offers a lot of options. You can go to a weekly meeting, weigh in, and talk with others on the same path. You can do everything from the comfort of your own home (or phone) instead. You can even meet with a diet coach if you want, share pictures from your journey with others online, and more.

Breakfast Recipes

Skinny One Point Weight Watcher Pancakes

Preparation + cooking time: 30 minutes

Servings: 14 pancakes

Ingredients

- 2 over-ripe bananas mashed
- 2 egg whites
- 1 cup of fat-free plain greek yogurt
- 1/2 cup of fat-free milk
- 1 teaspoon of pure vanilla extract
- 1 cup of all-purpose flour
- 2 teaspoons of baking powder
- 1/2 teaspoon of cinnamon

Instructions

1. Preheat a nonstick electric skillet to 325 degrees.
2. In a medium sized bowl, combine mashed bananas, egg whites, greek yogurt, milk and vanilla extract. Whisk until well combines.
3. In a larger bowl, combine flour, baking powder and cinnamon and whisk.
4. Stir wet ingredient into dry ingredients.
5. Pour 1/4 cup of batter onto hot skillet and cook until golden brown.

Recipe Notes
To make blueberry pancakes drop fresh blueberries into pancake batter once they are on the griddle.

Zero Point Muffin Tin Eggs

Preparation + cooking time: 50 minutes

Serves: 12

Ingredients
- 12 Eggs
- 1 teaspoon Montreal Steak Seasoning Blend
- 1 red, orange, or green pepper, diced
- ½ pound 99% fat-free ground turkey breast
- ½ teaspoon sage
- ½ teaspoon salt
- ½ teaspoon black pepper
- ¼ teaspoon red pepper flakes
- ¼ teaspoon marjoram
- Non-Stick Cooking Spray

Instructions
1. Preheat oven to 350 degrees.
2. Spray a muffin tin with non-stick spray.
3. Spray a large non-stick skillet with non-stick spray. On medium heat cook ground turkey, sage, salt, black pepper, red pepper flakes, and marjoram for 7-10 minutes or until cooked through. Stir consistently to prevent sticking.
4. While turkey is cooking, in a large bowl, beat eggs and Montreal steak seasoning together until well mixed and fluffy (2-3 minutes). Stir in diced bell pepper.
5. Once the turkey is cooked through, spoon into the muffin tins spreading equally between each muffin tin.
6. Pour egg mixture over the turkey filling ¾ of the way full. Bake at 350 degrees for 30 minutes.

Blueberry-Banana Bread

Ingredients:

- 3 large over-ripe bananas
- 2 tablespoons lemon juice
- 1/3 cup vanilla soymilk (or apple sauce)
- 1/2 cup agave nectar
- 2 cups white whole wheat flour,
- (or regular whole wheat flour)
- 3/4 teaspoon baking powder
- 3/4 teaspoon baking soda
- 1/2 teaspoon salt
- 1 cup blueberries

Directions:
1. Preheat oven to 350F. Spray or wipe a 9×5-inch loaf pan with oil (I used a silicon loaf pan).
2. Mix the soymilk with 1 tablespoon of the lemon juice and let stand until it curdles. (If using apple sauce, skip this step and add the lemon juice to the bananas.)
3. In a large bowl, mash the bananas and add the remaining lemon juice, soymilk, and agave nectar. Stir well to combine. In a separate bowl, combine the flour, baking powder, soda, and salt. Add the dry ingredients to the banana mixture, and stir just until the mixture is well-combined. Fold in the blueberries.
4. Spread the mixture evenly in the prepared pan and bake until a knife inserted in the center comes out clean, about 50-60 minutes. Allow to cool before cutting and serving. Cut into 12 E☐ual Slices
5. Makes 12 Servings (1 Slice Per Serving)

Avocado Toast with Sunny Side Egg

Preparation + cooking time: 30 minutes

Ingredients:
- slice whole grain bread, toasted (1.5 oz)
- 1 oz mashed (1/4 small haas) avocado
- cooking spray
- 1 large egg
- kosher salt and black pepper to taste hot sauce (optional)

Directions:
1. Mash the avocado in a small bowl and season with salt and pepper.
2. Heat a small nonstick skillet over low heat, spray with oil and gently crack the egg into the skillet. Cover and cook to your liking.
3. Place mashed avocado over toast, top with egg, salt and pepper and hot sauce if desired!

Avocado Veggie Egg Scramble

Preparation + cooking time: 20 minutes

Servings: 1-1.25 cups

Ingredients:
- 2 teaspoon olive oil
- 2 cups broccoli, chopped
- 1 red pepper, chopped
- 1/2 cup onion, diced
- 8 eggs, whisked
- Salt and pepper
- 1 tomato, diced
- 1 avocado

Directions:
1. Heat the olive oil over medium high heat.
2. Add the veggies and cook for 3-4 minutes until tender crisp.
3. Add the eggs and stir frequently to scramble to desired doneness.
4. Top with salt, pepper, diced tomato, and avocado.

Country Cottage Pancakes

Preparation + cooking time: 25 minutes

Servings: makes 18 medium pancakes

Ingredients:
- 1 cup / 7 oz / 200g cottage cheese
- 3/4 cup / 180 ml milk
- 4 room temperature eggs, separated
- 1 cup / 4 oz / 115g raw (or quickly blanched) cauliflower, chopped into rice-sized bits
- 1/2 cup / 75 g whole wheat pastry flour
- 1/2 cup / 75 g all-purpose flour
- 1 teaspoon baking powder scant
- 1/2 teaspoon fine grain sea salt butter, for cooking

Directions:
1. In a large bowl mix the cottage cheese, milk, and egg yolks until smooth. Stir in the cauliflower.
2. In a separate (clean) bowl, beat the egg whites until they hold stiff peaks.
3. Sift the flours, baking powder, and salt into another bowl. Add the flours to the cottage cheese mixture, and stir until just barely(!) combined. Gently fold the egg whites into the batter with a spatula. To cook, warm a griddle or pan over medium heat, melt a bit of butter in it, then spoon a little scoop (say, ~3 tablespoons) of batter into the pan for each pancake, working in batches.
4. You want to cook these relatively slowly, until each pancake is deeply golden on one side. Flip each pancake, and wait until the other side is golden, and the pancake is cooked through.

5. Continue until you've worked through all the batter. You can keep cooked pancakes in a 225F oven until you finish, to keep them warm.
6. They're great simply with a pat of butter and a sprinkling of salt. Or, if you want to get a bit fancy, whip up a bit of harissa, saffron or pesto- swirled salted yogurt.

Eggs Benedict Breakfast Flatbread

Preparation + cooking time: 15 minutes

Servings: makes for three servings

Ingredients:
- 2 Venice Bakery Flatbreads (They come in a pack of two)
- 4 eggs
- 4 slices of ham -or- Canadian bacon
- 3 egg yolks
- 1/2 cup butter
- 2 tablespoons lemon juice
- a dash of salt
- 1/2 teaspoon dried mustard
- a dash of hot sauce, or a pinch of cayenne pepper (optional)
- Separate the eggs and add to blender. Heat the butter in the microwave or on the stove, until steaming, but not boiling.
- With the blender turned on high, very slowly stream in the hot butter. Make sure the stream of butter is very small.

Directions:
1. Add lemon juice, salt, and optional hot sauce. Continue to blend until thick and creamy. Set aside.
2. Heat the oven to 500°.
3. Place your flatbreads on a baking stone or sheet and put in the oven for 3 minutes.
4. Pull out of the oven and top each piece of bread with a thick coating of the hollandaise sauce.
5. Arrange two slices of ham on each piece of flatbread.

6. Crack the eggs into a cup and slip them onto the pizza. Shake on a little salt and pepper and put back into the oven for another 5 minutes or until the yolk is just set and golden.

Mexican Chilaquiles

Preparation time + cooking time: 45 minutes

Servings: makes for four servings

Ingredients:
- 2 cups oil for frying
- 1/4 cup chopped onion
- 30 (6 inch) corn tortillas, torn into strips
- 6 eggs, lightly beaten
- 2 teaspoons salt
- 1 (7.75 ounce) can Mexican style hot tomato sauce
- 1/2 cup water
- 1/2 cup shredded Monterey Jack cheese

Directions:
1. In a large, heavy skillet, heat the oil to 350 degrees F (175 degrees C). Carefully stir in the onion and tortilla strips. Fry until tortilla strips are crisp and golden brown. Remove from heat, and drain on paper towels. Drain the skillet, leaving only a thin residue of oil.
2. Over medium heat, return tortillas to the skillet, and stir in the eggs. Season with salt. Cook and stir until eggs are firm.
3. Mix Mexican style hot tomato sauce and water into the skillet. Reduce heat, and simmer until thickened, about 10 minutes. Top with cheese. Continue cooking until cheese has melted.

Banana Oat Muffins

Preparation + Cooking Time: 35 minutes

Servings: makes twelve servings

Ingredients:
- 1/2 cups unbleached all-purpose flour
- 1 cup rolled oats
- 1/2 cup white sugar
- teaspoons baking powder
- 1 teaspoon baking soda
- 1/2 teaspoon salt
- 1 egg
- 3/4 cup milk
- 1/3 cup vegetable oil
- 1/2 teaspoon vanilla extract
- 1 cup mashed bananas

Directions:
1. Combine flour, oats, sugar, baking powder, soda, and salt. In a large bowl, beat the egg lightly.
2. Stir in the milk, oil, and vanilla.
3. Add the mashed banana, and combine thoroughly.
4. Stir the flour mixture into the banana mixture until just combined. Line a 12-cup muffin tin with paper bake cups, and divide the batter among them.
5. Bake at 400 degrees F (205 degrees C) for 18 to 20 minutes.

Peanut Butter and Jelly Yogurt Parfait Recipe

Preparation + cooking time: 8 minutes

Servings: makes four servings

Ingredients:
- 2 (6 oz) containers Yoplait Original French Vanilla Yogurt
- 6 tablespoons creamy peanut butter
- 1½ cups Nature Valley Protein Granola Peanut Butter
- 2 cups fresh strawberries, diced

Directions:
- Empty the yogurt into a medium bowl. Add the peanut butter and whisk until combined.
- Layer ⅛ of the yogurt mixture in the bottom of 4 (4 to 6-oz) jars or glasses.
- Sprinkle 3 tablespoons of granola over the yogurt in each glass, followed by ⅛ of the strawberries.
- Repeat the layers, using the remaining ingredients.
- Serve immediately.

Pumpkin Pie French Toast

Preparation + cooking time: 35 minutes

Servings: makes four servings

Ingredients:
- 3 large eggs
- 1/2 cup half-and-half cream
- 1/4 cup canned pumpkin puree
- 1 teaspoon ground cinnamon
- 1 teaspoon vanilla extract
- 1/4 teaspoon pumpkin pie spice
- 1/4 cup finely chopped walnuts
- 8 slices day-old bread

Directions:
1. Heat a lightly oiled skillet over medium heat.
2. Whisk eggs, half and half, pumpkin, cinnamon,
3. Vanilla extract, pumpkin pie spice, and walnuts together in a bowl.
4. Soak one slice of bread at a time in the pumpkin mixture, then place in the prepared skilled. Repeat with the remaining slices of bread.
5. Stir the pumpkin mixture between dips to keep the walnuts from settling.
6. Cook the bread until golden brown, about 3 minutes on each side.

Strawberry Banana Protein Smoothie

Preparation + cooking: 10 minutes

Servings: makes one serving

Ingredients:
- 1 banana
- 1 1/4 cups sliced fresh strawberries
- 10 whole almonds
- 2 tablespoons water
- 1 cup ice cubes
- 3 tablespoons chocolate flavored protein powder

Directions:
1. Place the banana, strawberries, almonds, and water into a blender.
2. Blend to mix, then add the ice cubes and puree until smooth.
3. Add the protein powder, and continue mixing until evenly incorporated, about 30 seconds.

Lunch

Mushroom Barley Soup

Preparation + cooking time: 1 hour 5 minutes

Servings: makes 6 servings

Ingredients:
- 1/4 cup olive oil
- 1 cup chopped onion
- 3/4 cup diced carrots
- 1/2 cup chopped celery
- 1 teaspoon minced garlic
- 1 pound sliced fresh mushrooms
- 6 cups chicken broth
- 3/4 cup barley salt and pepper to taste

Directions:
1. Heat the oil in a large soup pot over medium heat.
2. Add the onion, carrots, celery and garlic; cook and stir until onions are tender and transparent.
3. Stir in mushrooms and continue to cook for a few minutes.
4. Pour in the chicken broth and add barley.
5. Bring to a boil, then reduce heat to low.
6. Cover and simmer until barley is tender, about 50 minutes.
7. With salt and pepper before serving.

Quick and Easy Chicken Noodle Soup

Preparation + cooking time: 30 minutes

Servings: makes 6 servings

Ingredients:
- 1 tablespoon butter
- 1/2 cup chopped onion
- 1/2 cup chopped celery
- 4 (14.5 ounce) cans chicken broth
- 1 (14.5 ounce) can vegetable broth
- 1/2 pound chopped cooked chicken breast
- 1 1/2 cups egg noodles
- 1 cup sliced carrots
- 1/2 teaspoon dried basil
- 1/2 teaspoon dried oregano salt and pepper to taste

Directions:
1. In a large pot over medium heat, melt butter.
2. Cook onion and celery in butter until just tender, 5 minutes.
3. Pour in chicken and vegetable broths and stir in chicken, noodles, carrots, basil, oregano, salt and pepper.
4. Bring to a boil, then reduce heat and simmer 20 minutes before serving.

Smoked-Turkey and Fruit Wrap with Curried Aioli

Preparation + cooking time: 25 minutes

Servings: makes 4 servings

Ingredients:
- 1/2 cup mayonnaise
- 1 tablespoon minced garlic
- 1 teaspoon curry powder
- 4 (10-inch) flour tortillas
- 2 cups thinly sliced soft-leaf lettuce such as Boston (from 1 head)
- 1 medium sweet onion, halved lengthwise and thinly sliced crosswise
- 1 medium Granny Smith apple, cut into
- 1/4-inch-thick matchsticks
- 1 firm-ripe pear (preferably Anjou or Bosc), cut into 1/4-inch-thick matchsticks
- 1/2 pound thinly sliced smoked turkey

Directions:
1. Stir together mayonnaise, garlic, and curry powder to make aïoli. Lightly toast tortillas, 1 at a time, directly on burner (gas or electric) at moderately low heat, turning over once with tongs, until browned in spots but still flexible, about 30 seconds on each side.
2. Spread 2 tablespoons curried aïoli on each tortilla.
3. Divide lettuce, onion, apple, pear, and turkey among tortillas, layering them evenly.
4. Tightly roll up tortillas and cut in half diagonally.

The Ultimate Cuban Sandwich

Preparation + cooking time: 1 hour 24 minutes

Servings: makes 6 servings

Ingredients:
- 1-pound boneless pork shoulder
- Kosher salt and freshly ground black pepper
- 1 tablespoon ground cumin
- 1 tablespoon dried oregano
- 2 tablespoons extra-virgin olive oil
- 4 cloves garlic, peeled and gently smashed with the side of your knife
- 1/4 teaspoon dried red chili flakes
- 1 medium onion, sliced
- 1 cup fresh orange juice
- 1 lime, juiced
- 1 cup low-sodium chicken broth
- 2 bay leaves
- 1 long Cuban bread roll
- 3 tablespoons Dijon mustard
- 8 thin slices Swiss cheese
- 1 cup bread and butter pickles
- 8 thin slices deli ham
- Olive oil

Directions:
1. Begin by braising the pork shoulder.
2. Tie the shoulder in 4 places with kitchen twine so it will hold its shape while being cooked or ask your butcher to do this for you.
3. Season the pork with salt, pepper, cumin and oregano.
4. Set the base of a pressure cooker over low-medium heat and add a 2 count of olive oil.

5. Add garlic and chili flakes and as the oil heats up it will become fragrant and infuse the oil.
6. Add the pork.
7. Add onions around the pork and brown slightly before adding orange juice, lime juice, stock and bay leaves.
8. Secure the lid of the pressure cooker and cook for 20 to 25 minutes depending on the size of your pressure cooker.
9. The pork should be tender when done. When done allow to cool in juices before removing twine and slicing.
10. To prepare Cuban sandwiches, split bread in half then layer the sandwich with mustard, cheese, pickles, ham, pork then cheese again (the cheese glues everything together).
11. Season with salt and pepper in between the ham and pork layers. (Optional: drizzle a little of the pork braising liquid over the meat as well).
12. To cook, heat a large cast iron skillet or grill pan over medium heat and lightly coat with olive oil. Place the sandwiches on the skillet and top with another heavy skillet and a couple of heavy weights (bricks, or cans of tomatoes work well).
13. Press down firmly and cook for 5 to 7 minutes per side until the sandwich has compressed to about a third of its original size and the bread is super-crispy.
14. Serve with beans, rice and plantain chips.

Green Bloody Mary

Preparation + cooking time: 10 minutes

Servings: makes 4 servings

Ingredients:
- 6 ounces' vodka
- Green Bloody Mary Mix
- 5 tomatillos husks removed
- 3 medium yellow tomatoes
- 2 stalks celery
- 1 jalapeno
- 3 tablespoons chopped cilantro
- 1 1/2 cups water
- 1 1/2 teaspoons horseradish
- 1/4 teaspoon cumin
- 1/2 teaspoon salt
- 1/4 teaspoon pepper GARNISH
- Celery
- Golden tomatoes
- Serrano peppers
- Salt & Chili Powder

Directions:

GREEN BLOODY MARY MIX

1. Cut the tomatoes, tomatillos, celery and jalapeno into large chunks. Add to your blender along with chopped cilantro, horseradish, water and spices.
2. Process until smooth.
3. Taste and adjust your seasonings as desired.
4. If you prefer a thinner bloody mary, strain the mixture through a fine mesh strainer.
5. For a thicker cocktail, serve as is.
6. I prefer to strain half of my mixture and then combine it with the thick, for a medium consistency.

7. Chill before serving.

TO SERVE

1. To rim your glass, combine a mixture of 1/2 kosher salt and 1/2 chili powder in a small rimmed dish. Run a lemon around the lip of your glass and then dip it into the salt to coat.
2. Add 1-1/2 ounces' vodka to your glass and top with the bloody Mary mix.
3. Garnish with a celery stick and skewered tomatoes.

Smoked Salmon Canapés with Cream Cheese

Preparation + cooking time: 45 minutes

Servings: makes 6 servings

Ingredients:
- Rye crisp breads
- 1 tub of cream cheese
- 2 tablespoons creme fraiche
- 2 large unwaxed lemons (juice and zest of 1.5)
- 1 large bunch of dill, part chopped finely, part sprigs reserved Freshly milled black pepper

Directions:
1. Mix the cream cheese, crème fraîche, chopped dill, lemon juice and half the zest, then add freshly milled black pepper.
2. Place the crisp breads on serving trays.
3. Scoop some cream cheese filling and place on top of each of the crisp breads, using a fork to make the swirls.
4. Cut the smoked salmon slices into ribbons, then roll and twist, and place on top of the crisp breads.
5. Top with individual sprigs of dill. Garnish with a couple of strands of the lemon zest.

Italian Chicken Salad

Preparation + cooking time: 20 minutes

Servings: makes 4 servings

Ingredients:

- ✓ DRESSING
- 1tablespoon olive oil
- 1tablespoon lemon juice
- 1tablespoon red wine vinegar
- 1/2teaspoon garlic, minced
- 1/2teaspoon sugar
- 1/4teaspoon fresh ground black pepper
- 1/8teaspoon salt

- ✓ SALAD
- 3cups chicken breasts, cooked and cubed
- 1cup red bell pepper, finely chopped
- 2tablespoons fresh parsley, finely chopped
- 1teaspoon dried oregano
- 1/2teaspoon dried basil
- 10pitted ripe olives, halved
- 1(14 ounce) can quartered artichoke hearts, drained

Directions:
1. DRESSING: Combine all dressing ingredients in a medium bowl, stirring with a whisk.
2. SALAD: Combine chicken and remaining ingredients in a large bowl.
3. Pour dressing over salad, and toss gently to combine.

Garlic Shrimp and Zucchini Salad

Preparation + cooking time: 25 minutes

Servings: makes 4 servings

Ingredients:
- 1cup panko bread crumbs
- 2 cloves garlic, finely chopped
- 1 tsp. salt
- 1/4 cup olive oil
- lb. shrimp, peeled

Directions:
1. Preheat the broiler. Stir together the panko, garlic, and salt in a large bowl.
2. Drizzle in the olive oil and stir to combine.
3. Toss the shrimp in the panko mixture, using your hands to gently press it into each shrimp.
4. Move the shrimp to a baking sheet and top with any panko that didn't stick to the shrimp.
5. Place the baking sheet under the broiler until the shrimp are cooked on one side, about 3-5 minutes depending on the size of the shrimp and heat of the broiler.
6. Flip the shrimp and broil on the second side.
7. Serve shrimp and any loose pieces of cooked panko over raw zucchini salad; recipe below.

Crab, Mango and Chili Salad

Preparation + cooking time: 10 minutes

Servings: makes 4 servings

Ingredients:
- 2tablespoons lime juice
- 1 teaspoons fish sauce
- 1 whole fresh red chili, deseeded, finely chopped
- 350 g Crab, boiled or steamed, (crab meat)
- 1/4 cup(s) fresh mint, leaves
- 1/4 cup(s) fresh coriander, leaves
- 2 medium Lebanese cucumber, cut into ribbons
- 1 small red onion, thinly sliced
- 200 g Tomato, yellow grape tomatoes, halved
- 100 g coral lettuce, mixed lettuce leaves
- 2 medium mangoes, cut into cheeks

Directions:
1. To make dressing, combine lime juice, fish sauce and chilli in a medium bowl, then add fresh crab meat, mint and coriander.
2. In a large bowl, toss cucumber, onion, tomatoes and lettuce, then top with the crab mixture and peeled mango cheeks.
3. Serve immediately.

Lentil Salad with Poached Eggs

Preparation + cooking time: 30 minutes

Servings: makes 4 servings

Ingredients:
- 250 g cherry tomato
- 1 cup(s) Dry lentils, (200g), French-style green variety
- 100 g Mushrooms, button variety, sliced
- 2 tablespoons reduced-fat French dressing
- 60 g baby spinach leaves
- 3 individual Green shallots, thinly sliced
- 4 medium egg(s)

Directions:
1. Preheat oven to 180°C or 160°C fan-forced. Line a baking tray with baking paper.
2. Place tomatoes on prepared tray and bake for 20 minutes or until soft. Cool slightly.
3. Meanwhile, cook lentils in a large saucepan of boiling water, following packet instructions, until just tender.
4. Drain. Transfer to a large bowl. Add tomatoes, mushrooms, dressing, spinach and shallots and toss to combine. Season with salt and pepper. Half-fill a medium frying pan with water and heat over medium-high heat until just simmering.
5. Crack 1 egg into a cup, and then carefully slide egg into the pan. Cook for 3 minutes or until white has set but yolk is still soft. Using a slotted spoon, transfer to a plate.
6. Repeat with remaining eggs (you can cook several at once to save time).
7. Top lentil salad with eggs and sprinkle with pepper to serve.

Smashed Bean, Tomato and Feta Wrap

Preparation + cooking time: 5 minutes

Servings: makes 4 servings

Ingredients:
- 1 can(s) Canned mixed beans, (1x300g can) rinsed, drained
- 1 large Tomato, coarsely chopped
- 6 individual black olives, drained, kalamata variety, thinly sliced
- 25 g reduced fat feta cheese, crumbled
- 1 tsp lemon juice
- 80 g Wholegrain wrap, (2x40g)
- 3 cup(s) cos lettuce, (6 baby cos leaves)

Directions:
1. Place beans in a medium bowl and mash with a fork.
2. Add tomato, olives, feta and juice and stir to combine.
3. Season with pepper.
4. Top wraps with bean mixture and lettuce. Roll tightly to enclose filling. Serve.

Dinner

Slow Cooker Shredded Korean Pork

Preparation + cooking time: 8 hours 10 minutes

Servings: makes 8 servings

Ingredients:
- 3 lb lean pork tenderloin
- 1/3 cup brown sugar (or Stevia)
- 1/3 cup low sodium soy sauce
- 10 cloves garlic, whole
- 1/2 cup red onion, diced
- 2 jalapenos, diced (or substitute 2-4 tablespoons Sriracha)
- 2 tablespoons fresh ginger root, peeled and grated
- 1 tablespoon rice wine vinegar
- 2 tablespoons sesame seeds

Directions:
1. Combine the sugar, soy sauce, red onion, jalapenos, ginger, rice vinegar, sesame seeds in a small bowl.
2. Add the pork and garlic to the crock pot and cover with the sauce. Cook for 8 hours on low.
3. When it has 30 minutes left to cook and the pork can be easily shredded with a fork, break it into larger pieces.
4. Continue cooking without the lid on so the sauce thickens up. Finish shredding the pork.

Spring Rolls

Preparation + cooking time: 30 minutes

Servings: makes 8 servings

Ingredients:
- 10 oz firm tofu, drained well
- 8 rice paper spring roll wrappers
- 1 carrot, thinly sliced
- 1 cucumber, thinly sliced
- 1 cup lettuce
- 1 cup red cabbage, shredded
- 1/8 cup fresh cilantro
- 1/8 cup basil
- 1/8 cup mint
- 3 tablespoon fat free chicken broth (for sauce)
- 2.5 tablespoons peanut butter (for sauce)
- 1 tablespoon low sodium soy sauce (for sauce, or coconut aminos)
- 1/2 tablespoon lime juice (for sauce)
- 2 tsp honey (for sauce)
- 1 teaspoon red curry paste (for sauce)

Directions:
1. Prepare all the ingredients. Cut the tofu into thin rectangles.
2. To make the spring rolls, submerge one piece of rice paper into water for 15-20 seconds.
3. Remove and place on a damp cloth. Place the tofu in the center of the paper.
4. Layer on the vegetables and herbs.
5. Carefully fold over one end and then fold over the sides. Then roll over carefully to close the spring roll.

6. Normally there are directions on the rice paper package for rolling. Make the peanut sauce by combining the chicken broth, peanut butter, soy sauce, lime juice, curry paste, and honey.
7. Serve the spring rolls with the peanut sauce.

Slow Cooker Cheesy Southwestern Chicken

Preparation + cooking time: 3 hours 10 minutes

Servings: makes 6 servings

Ingredients:
- 30 oz. canned corn, drained
- 15 oz. canned black beans, rinsed and drained
- 16 oz. thick and chunky salsa, divided
- 2 lb. boneless skinless chicken breast
- 1 tablespoon taco seasoning (optional, or Southwestern seasoning)
- 1 cup reduced fat shredded
- Mexican cheese blend

Directions:
1. Ideal slow cooker size: 5- to 6-Quart.
2. Combine the corn, black beans and 1/2 cup salsa in the slow cooker. Season the chicken with Southwest seasoning blend (if using) or salt and pepper to taste.
3. Add chicken to the slow cooker. Top with the remaining salsa.
4. Cover and cook on LOW for 4 to 6 hours, or until chicken is tender. Sprinkle with cheese. Cover and cook 5 minutes more or until cheese melts.

Cajun Salmon

Preparation + cooking time: 15 minutes

Servings: makes 4 servings

Ingredients:
- 1.33 lbs salmon
- 1 tablespoon olive oil
- 2 tsp paprika
- 1/2 tsp garlic powder
- 1/2 tsp onion powder
- 1/2 tsp salt
- 1/2 tsp pepper
- 1/4 tsp dried thyme
- 1/8 tsp cayenne (adjust to preference)

Directions:
Mix together the spices to create the Cajun seasoning. Brush the salmon with the olive oil and coat the flesh side in the seasoning.

Broiler: Preheat the broiler with an oven rack about 6 inches away from the heat.
Place the salmon on a baking sheet, lined with foil for easier clean up. Broil for 6-8 minutes until is just cooked through and flaky.

Grill: Place the salmon skin side down on to a hot grill.
Cook for 3-4 minutes until almost cooked through. Flip and cook for 1- 3 minutes until cooked to your liking.

Pan Seared: Heat a cast iron skillet or heavy bottom pan over medium high heat.

Add the fish, skin side down, and cook for about 3-4 minutes until the fish is almost cooked through.
Flip and cook for 1-2 minutes until fish is cooked to your liking.

Baked: Preheat the oven to 400 degrees. Bake for 10-12 minutes until cooked to your liking.

Thai Chicken Skewers

Ingredients:

- 1.33 lbs boneless skinless chicken breast, chopped
- 1/2 cup nonfat Greek yogurt (or canned coconut milk for Paleo)
- 2 tablespoons cilantro
- 1 tablespoon red curry paste
- 1 tablespoon low sodium soy sauce (or coconut aminos for Paleo, GF)
- 1 tablespoon lime juice
- 1 tablespoon honey (leave out for low carb, or Stevia)
- 1/4 cup fat free chicken broth (for sauce)
- 3 tablespoons peanut butter (for sauce)
- 1 tablespoon low sodium soy sauce (for sauce, or coconut aminos)
- 1/2 tablespoon lime juice (for sauce)
- 2 tsp honey (for sauce)
- 1 tsp red curry paste (for sauce)

Directions:

1. Combine the yogurt, cilantro, curry paste, soy sauce, lime juice, honey, and turmeric.
2. Marinate the chicken in this mixture for at least 4 hours, ideally overnight.
3. When ready to cook, thread the chicken on skewers, letting excess marinade drip off.
4. Grill for 3-4 minutes per side until cooked through.
5. Make the peanut sauce by combining the chicken broth, peanut butter, soy sauce, lime juice, curry paste, and honey.
6. Serve the skewers with the peanut sauce drizzled on top or on the side. Broiling option: Place the chicken skewers on a baking sheet covered in foil. Broil for 3-4 minutes on each side until chicken is cooked through.

Skinny Chicken Alfredo Pizza

Preparation + cooking time: 27 minutes

Servings: makes 1 serving

Ingredients:
- 1/2 cup self-rising flour (see picture)
- 1/2 cup nonfat plain Greek yogurt
- 1 teaspoon light butter, melted
- 2 tablespoons skim milk
- 1/4 teaspoon garlic powder
- 1 tablespoon Parmesan cheese
- Salt and pepper
- 3 tablespoons nonfat plain Greek yogurt
- 4 oz cooked chicken breast, shredded
- 1 cup fresh spinach
- 1/4 cup shredded asiago cheese

Directions:
1. Preheat oven to 375F
2. Make your dough by mixing your ½ cup of flour with ½ cup of yogurt. Sprinkle a little flour on flat surface and knead dough for 2 minutes.
3. Roll out dough on a sprayed piece of parchment paper, I made my crust more on the thin side for this pizza.
4. Pre-bake dough in oven for 12 minutes.
5. Now make your Alfredo sauce, melt your 1 teaspoon butter in the microwave, 10-15 seconds should do it. Stir in your milk and your garlic powder, return to microwave and heat for 30 seconds. Then stir in your parmesan cheese, salt & pepper, and whisk in yogurt. It should give you a creamy sauce.

6. Spread sauce over your pre-baked pizza dough leaving the edges clear. Top with your spinach, shredded chicken, asiago cheese, and seasoning.
7. Bake in the oven for approximately for 14-16 minutes.
8. Serve immediately, I cut mine into 6 pieces, on WW freestyle the whole pizza is 9.

Roasted Cauliflower Steaks

Preparation + cooking time: 30 minutes

Servings: makes 4 servings

Ingredients:
- 1 large cauliflowers
- 1 tablespoon olive oil Salt and pepper
- 3 tablespoons parsley, minced
- 3 tablespoons cilantro, minced
- 1 clove garlic, minced
- 2 tablespoons olive oil
- 1 tablespoon red wine vinegar
- 1 tablespoon water
- 1/4 teaspoon kosher salt
- 1/8 teaspoon black pepper
- 1/8 teaspoon red pepper flakes

Directions:
1. Preheat the oven to 400 degrees.
2. Remove the green stems around the base of the cauliflower.
3. Slice the cauliflower in half. Moving away from the center, cut the cauliflower into steaks. You should be able to get four steaks from a large cauliflower.
4. You will have some extra cauliflower left. You can save it or roast it alongside the steaks.
5. Brush the steaks with olive oil on both sides and sprinkle with salt and pepper. Place on a baking sheet.
6. Bake for 20-25 minutes, carefully flipping halfway through so they brown on both sides.

7. Meanwhile make the chimichurri by combining the remaining ingredients. This can be done by hand or in a food processor if you don't want to mince the herbs and garlic.
8. Serve the cauliflower steaks with the chimichurri drizzled on top.

Healthy Eggplant Parmesan

Preparation + cooking time: 55 minutes

Servings: makes 4 servings

Ingredients:
- 1 tablespoon. olive oil
- 2 medium eggplants, cut into rounds
- 2 tseaspoons Italian seasoning
- 1/2 cup seasoned breadcrumbs
- 16 oz. marinara sauce (look for low sugar)
- 1 cup reduced fat mozzarella cheese
- 1/4 cup fresh basil

Directions:
1. Preheat the oven to 400 degrees.
2. Cover 2 baking sheets with foil and spray with cooking spray.
3. Place the eggplant in a single layer on the baking sheets. Brush with olive oil. Sprinkle with salt, pepper, and Italian seasoning.
4. Then sprinkle breadcrumbs on top. Bake for 20-25 minutes until softened.
5. Meanwhile, coat an 8 X 8 glass baking dish with cooking spray. Add about 1/3 of the sauce to the bottom.
6. Add a layer of the baked eggplant. Sprinkle with 1/2 the cheese.
7. Add more sauce, another layer of eggplant, more sauce, and then sprinkle the remaining cheese on top.
8. Cover with foil and bake for 20 minutes. Remove foil and let cheese brown if desired.
9. Serve with fresh basil.

Black Bean and Corn Quesadillas - Freezer Friendly

Preparation + cooking time: 15 minutes

Servings: makes 4 servings

Ingredients:
- 2 teaspoon olive oil
- 1/2 red onion, diced
- 1 garlic clove, minced
- 15 oz. canned black beans, rinsed and drained
- 15 oz. canned corn, rinsed and drained
- 1 tomato, diced (or 1/2 cup salsa)
- 2 tsp. taco seasoning (store bought or homemade)
- 1 cup reduced fat shredded cheddar cheese (any cheese works)
- 8 low carb tortillas
- Cooking spray

Directions:
1. Heat the olive oil in a pan over medium high heat. Add the onion and cook for 5-8 minutes, until softened.
2. Add the garlic and cook for 30 seconds.
3. Mix together the onion, garlic, black beans, corn, tomatoes, taco seasoning, and cheese
4. Spray a pan with cooking spray. Add one tortilla and gently add the filling.
5. Top with another tortilla. Cook until the tortilla begins to brown and cheese is melting.
6. Carefully flip and cook on the other side. Repeat with remaining tortillas.

Roasted Chicken and Potatoes with Broccoli

Preparation + cooking time: 35 minutes

Servings: makes 4 servings

Ingredients:
- 1/3 cup fat free chicken broth
- 2 tablespoons butter, melted
- 3 cloves garlic, minced
- 1 tablespoons Italian seasoning
- 1.33 lbs boneless skinless chicken (cut into cutlets)
- 1 lb potatoes, cut into wedges
- 1 lb broccoli

Directions:
1. Preheat the oven to 425 degrees.
2. Mix together the chicken broth, melted butter, garlic, and Italian seasoning.
3. Carefully cut the potato into wedges.
4. Cut the potato in half and then cut each half into 4-5 wedges. This ensures they will cook fully.
5. Toss with half of the chicken broth and butter mixture.
6. Spread out onto a baking sheet, sprayed with cooking spray, in a single layer. Season with salt and pepper.
7. Place in the oven for 15 minutes.
8. While the potatoes cook, toss the chicken and broccoli with the remaining chicken broth and butter mixture.
9. If you have large chicken breasts, cut them in half horizontally so that they will cook in the allotted time.
10. Remove the sheet pan from the oven.
11. Carefully push the potatoes to one side. Usually, I flip them at this point.
12. Add the chicken and broccoli to the pan.
13. Season with salt and pepper.

14. Return to the oven and cook for 12-15 minutes until everything is fully cooked.

Snacks

Brownie Batter Dip

Preparation + cooking time: 5 minutes

Servings: 30

Ingredients:
- 8 oz cream cheese
- 8 oz cool whip
- 1 - 18. 4 oz box brownie mix (dry)
- 2 TBS cocoa powder
- 1/4 cup milk
- 1 cup mini chocolate chips (optional)

Directions:
1. Combine your cream cheese, cool whip, brownie mix, cocoa powder and milk in a large bowl.
2. Stir until everything is creamy and combined.
3. Mix in chocolate chips if desired, and sprinkle some on top for decoration too.
4. Serve with whatever you want to dip in it - cookies, pretzels, fruit and more.

Caramel Pretzel Bites Recipe

Preparation + cooking time: 45 minutes

Servings: makes 72 servings

Ingredients:
- 2 teaspoons butter, softened
- 4 cups pretzel sticks
- 2-1/2 cups pecan halves, toasted
- 2-1/4 cups packed brown sugar
- 1 cup butter, cubed
- 1 cup corn syrup
- 1 can (14 ounces) sweetened condensed milk
- 1/8 teaspoon salt
- 1 teaspoon vanilla extract
- 1 package (11-1/2 ounces) milk chocolate chips
- 1 tablespoon plus
- 1 teaspoon shortening, divided
- 1/3 cup white baking chips

Directions:
1. Line a 13x9-in. pan with foil; grease foil with softened butter. Spread pretzels and pecans on bottom of prepared pan.
2. In a large heavy saucepan, combine brown sugar, cubed butter, corn syrup, milk and salt; cook and stir over medium heat until a candy thermometer reads 240° (soft-ball stage). Remove from heat. Stir in vanilla. Pour over pretzel mixture.
3. In a microwave, melt chocolate chips and 1 tablespoon shortening; stir until smooth.

4. Spread over caramel layer. In microwave, melt white baking chips and remaining shortening; stir until smooth. Drizzle over top. Let stand until set.
5. Using foil, lift candy out of pan; remove foil. Using a buttered knife, cut candy into bite-size pieces.

Crunchy Spiced Chickpeas

Preparation + cooking time: 1 hour 10 minutes

Servings: makes four servings

Ingredients:
- 1 cup dried chickpeas (garbanzo beans)
- 2 tablespoons olive oil
- 1 pinch ground cumin, or to taste
- 1 pinch paprika, or to taste
- 1 pinch cayenne pepper, or to taste
- salt and freshly ground black pepper to taste

Directions:
1. Place chickpeas in a large container and cover with several inches of cool water; let stand for 24 hours.
2. Drain and dry on paper towels.
3. Preheat oven to 400 degrees F (200 degrees C).
4. Pour chickpeas into a baking dish; drizzle olive oil over the top and season with cumin, paprika, cayenne pepper, salt, and black pepper.
5. Stir to coat chickpeas.
6. Bake in the preheated oven, stirring every 20 minutes, until crispy and fragrant, about 1 hour.
7. Transfer to a wire rack to cool completely.

Frozen Yogurt Buttons

Preparation + cooking time: 1 hour 5 minutes

Servings: makes one serving

Ingredients:
- 1-100g yogurt container of choice (Greek or regular)
- Sprinkles

Directions:
1. Spoon your yogurt into a small zip lock bag and cut a small hole in the corner of bag.
2. Pipe onto a cookie sheet into button shapes.
3. Sprinkle your candy sprinkles on top (or topping of choice) Freeze for at least an hour, store in freezer until ready to eat. The yogurt is a Canadian brand (Skyr by PC) and is only 1SP for the
4. amount being used, in the U.S I would suggest the Dannon light and fit. You could use about ½T sprinkles so your bowl of buttons is only 1sp/pp, points will depend on yogurt brand and your topping. Of course these will melt over time, so you can't just leave them sitting there, but they do last awhile before melting.

Fried Mozzarella Cheese Sticks

Preparation time + cooking time: 30 minutes

Servings: makes eight servings

Ingredients:
- 2 eggs, beaten
- 1/4 cup water
- 1 1/2 cups Italian seasoned bread crumbs
- 1/2 teaspoon garlic salt
- 2/3 cup all-purpose flour
- 1/3 cup cornstarch
- 1-quart oil for deep frying
- 1 (16 ounce) package mozzarella cheese sticks

Directions:
1. In a small bowl, mix the eggs and water.
2. Mix the bread crumbs and garlic salt in a medium bowl. In a medium bowl, blend the flour and cornstarch.
3. In a large heavy saucepan, heat the oil to 365 degrees F (185 degrees C).
4. One at a time, coat each mozzarella stick in the flour mixture, then the egg mixture, then in the bread crumbs and finally into the oil.
5. Fry until golden brown, about 30 seconds.
6. Remove from heat and drain on paper towels.

Greek-Style Nachos

Preparation time + cooking time: 40 minutes

Servings: makes four servings

Ingredients:
- 2 tablespoons olive oil, plus extra to brush
- 1 small onion, chopped
- 2 garlic cloves, chopped
- 1 tablespoons tomato paste
- 500g lamb mince
- 2 tablespoons chopped oregano leaves
- 4 thin pita breads, cut into triangles
- 2 red capsicums, thinly sliced
- 2/3 cup (100g) pitted kalamata olives
- 1/3 cup (50g) pine nuts, toasted
- 1/2 bunch mint, leaves picked Tzatziki
- 1 cup (280g) thick Greek-style yoghurt
- 1 garlic clove, crushed
- 1 Lebanese cucumber, finely chopped
- 1 tablespoon olive oil
- 1/2 bunch mint, leaves picked
- Finely grated zest of 1 lemon

Directions:
1. Preheat the oven to 200C.
2. Heat oil in a saucepan over medium heat. Add onion and cook, stirring, for 2 minutes or until softened. Add the garlic and cook, stirring, for 1 minute.
3. Add tomato paste and cook, stirring, for a further 2 minutes, then add the mince, oregano and 1/3 cup (80ml) hot water. Season, then cook for 15 minutes or until reduced.

4. Meanwhile, brush pita bread triangles with a little oil and place on a baking tray.
5. Bake for 10 minutes or until golden.
6. For the tzatziki, combine all the ingredients in a bowl and set aside.
7. To serve, place the pita chips on a plate and top with mince, tzatziki, capsicum, olives, pine nuts and mint leaves.

Hawaiian Pizza Cups

Preparation + cooking time: 35 minutes

Servings: makes 20 servings

Ingredients:
- 2 cans Pillsbury refrigerated biscuits 10 biscuits each can
- 2 cups spaghetti sauce your favorite flavor
- 3/4 to 1 cup diced ham
- 1/2 to 2/3 cup diced pineapple
- 1/3 cup finely diced green bell pepper
- shredded Mozzarella cheese

Directions:
1. Spray 20 muffin tins with cooking spray.
2. Spread biscuits and stretch them into the muffin tins as well as possible to cover the bottom and sides.
3. Spoon 1 HEAPING tablespoon spaghetti sauce into each biscuit. Place about three pieces each of ham and pineapple on top of sauce. Sprinkle 3-4 pieces' green pepper over top of ham.
4. Sprinkle mozzarella cheese over top of each muffin tin.
5. Bake at 400° about 15-20 minutes until cheese melts and biscuits are lightly browned.
6. Do not overbake.
7. Allow to cool a minute or two before removing pizza cups from muffin tins.
8. Serve.

Homestyle Potato Chips

Preparation + cooking time: 60 minutes

Servings: makes 8 servings

Ingredients:
- 4 medium potatoes, peeled and sliced paper-thin
- 3 tablespoons salt
- 1-quart oil for deep frying

Directions:
1. Place potato slices into a large bowl of cold water as you slice. Drain, and rinse, then refill the bowl with water, and add the salt.
2. Let the potatoes soak in the salty water for at least 30 minutes. Drain, then rinse and drain again.
3. Heat oil in a deep-fryer to 365 degrees F (185 degrees C).
4. Fry potato slices in small batches. Once they start turning golden, remove and drain on paper towels.
5. Continue until all of the slices are fried. Season with additional salt if desired.

Dessert

Coconut and Almond Macaroons

Preparation time + cooking time: 45 minutes
Servings: makes 18 servings
Ingredients:
- 2 egg whites
- 115g (4 oz) icing sugar
- 115g (4 oz) ground almonds
- 1/4 teaspoon vanilla extract
- 115g (4 oz) dessicated coconut

Directions:
1. Preheat the oven to 150 degrees C (Gas 2). Grease two baking trays.
2. Use an electric beater to whisk the egg whites until stiff but moist.
3. Sift in the icing sugar and gently fold into the egg whites.
4. Gently fold in the almonds, vanilla extract and dessicated coconut until the mixture is combined, forming a sticky dough.
5. Spoon walnut-sized pieces of the mixture onto the baking trays.
6. Bake in the oven for 20-25 minutes, until the macaroons are crisp and golden on the outside.
7. Transfer to a cooling rack.

Missy's Lemon and Blueberry Cupcakes

Preparation + cooking time: 40 minutes

Servings: makes 12 cakes

Ingredients:

Batter
- 1 1/2 sticks unsalted butter (let stand at room temperature)
- 3 eggs (let stand at room temperature)
- 1 3/4 cups all-purpose flour
- 1/4 teaspoon baking powder
- 1/4 teaspoon baking soda
- 1/4 teaspoon salt
- 1 1/4 cups granulated sugar
- 1/4 cup milk
- 3 tablespoons finely shredded lemon peel
- Butter baking spray
- Blueberries, coated with flour

Frosting:
- 3 to 4 cups powdered sugar
- 1 stick unsalted butter (let stand at room temperature)
- 1 stick cream cheese
- 2 tablespoons fresh lemon juice
- 2 tablespoons lemon zest

Decoration:
- Lemon peel
- Blueberries
- Sprig of fresh mint

Directions:
1. Preheat the oven to 350 degrees F.
2. For the batter: Mix the butter and eggs.
3. In a medium bowl, mix the flour, baking powder, baking soda and salt together.
4. Mix the granulated sugar, milk and lemon peel together. Then mix the butter and eggs into the milk and sugar mixture. Mix the flour into the wet mixture and blend.
5. Place paper cups into a pan, spray with butter baking spray and fill each cup three-quarters full with batter.
6. Drop the coated blueberries on top. Bake for 18 to 20 minutes.
7. For the frosting: Combine the powdered sugar, butter, cream cheese, lemon juice and zest together until light and fluffy.
8. Pipe onto the cupcakes and decorate with lemon peel, blueberries and a mint leaf.

Chocolate Covered Strawberries

Preparation + cooking: 50 minutes

Servings: makes 1-pound chocolate covered strawberries

Ingredients:
- 6 ounces' semisweet chocolate, chopped
- 3 ounces' white chocolate, chopped
- 1 pound strawberries with stems (about 20), washed and dried very well

Directions:
1. Put the semisweet and white chocolates into 2 separate heatproof medium bowls.
2. Fill 2 medium saucepans with a couple inches of water and bring to a simmer over medium heat.
3. Turn off the heat; set the bowls of chocolate over the water to melt.
4. Stir until smooth, (Alternatively, melt the chocolates in a microwave at half power, for 1 minute, stir and then heat for another minute or until melted.)
5. Once the chocolates are melted and smooth, remove from the heat. Line a sheet pan with parchment or waxed paper.
6. Holding the strawberry by the stem, dip the fruit into the dark chocolate, lift and twist slightly, letting any excess chocolate fall back into the bowl.
7. Set strawberries on the parchment paper. Repeat with the rest of the strawberries.
8. Dip a fork in the white chocolate and drizzle the white chocolate over the dipped strawberries.
9. Set the strawberries aside until the chocolate sets, about 30 minutes.

Baked French Toast Muffins

Preparation + cooking time: 40 minutes

Servings: makes 12 muffins

Ingredients:

For the Muffins:
- 1 loaf French bread, cut or torn into
- 1/2 inch cubes (about 12 cups of bread)
- 2 1/2 cups milk
- 6 large eggs
- 1/2 cup granulated sugar
- 1 tablespoon vanilla extract
- 1 teaspoon ground cinnamon

For the Cinnamon Streusel Topping:
- 1/4 cup cold butter
- 1/4 cup light brown sugar
- 1/4 cup all-purpose flour
- 1/8 teaspoon ground cinnamon
- Pinch of salt
- Butter and Maple Syrup, for serving, optional

Directions:
1. In a medium bowl, whisk together the milk, eggs, sugar, vanilla, and cinnamon.
2. Grease a 12 cup muffin tin. Add about 1 cup of bread cubes to each muffin cup.
3. Carefully pour egg and milk mixture evenly over each muffin tin.
4. You may need to press down on the bread cubes after you pour a little mixture and then pour more. Pour slowly or you will have a mess.

5. Or you can combine everything in a large bowl and then fill the muffin cups.
6. Cover the muffins with plastic wrap and refrigerate for 2 hours or up to overnight.
7. When ready to bake, preheat the oven to 350 degrees F.
8. To make the cinnamon streusel, in a small bowl, combine butter, brown sugar, flour, cinnamon, and salt.
9. Mix together with your hands, until you have a crumbly mixture.
10. Remove the muffins from the refrigerator and sprinkle the muffins evenly with the streusel topping.
11. Bake for 25 minutes or until tops are golden brown.
12. Let muffins cool for 5 minutes. Remove from pan and serve with butter and maple syrup, if desired.

Easy Swedish Meatball Sauce

Preparation + cooking time: 20 minutes

Servings: makes 4 servings

Ingredients:
- 1 cup beef stock
- 1 cup heavy cream
- 3 tablespoons all-purpose flour
- 1 tablespoon soy sauce
- 1 teaspoon ground black pepper
- 1/2 teaspoon dried rosemary
- 1/2 (20 ounce) package frozen cooked meatballs, thawed

Directions:
1. Whisk together the beef stock, heavy cream, flour, soy sauce, black pepper, and rosemary in a large saucepan until smooth.
2. Cook and stir over low heat until thickened, about 10 minutes, stirring occasionally.
3. Stir in the meatballs, and continue cooking until meatballs are heated through, about 5 more minutes.

Honey Mustard Glazed Ham

Preparation + cooking time: 2 hours 10 minutes

Servings: makes 8-10 servings

Ingredients:
- One 9-pound bone-in spiral-sliced ham
- 1 cup honey
- 1/3 cup brown sugar
- 4 tablespoons unsalted butter
- 3 tablespoons Dijon mustard
- 2 tablespoons whole-grain mustard
- 2 teaspoons finely chopped fresh thyme

Directions:
1. Preheat the oven to 325 degrees F.
2. Place the ham in a small roasting pan, cut-side down, and pour 1/2 cup water into the bottom of the pan.
3. Cover the pan tightly with foil.
4. Bake until the ham is heated through, about 1 1/2 hours.
5. Meanwhile, combine the honey, brown sugar, butter, Dijon mustard, whole-grain mustard and thyme in a small saucepan.
6. Cook over medium-low heat until the sugar has dissolved, about 2 minutes.
7. Increase the oven temperature to 375 degrees F.
8. While the ham is still hot, remove the foil and carefully pour off the water from the roasting pan; it is fine if a little water remains.
9. Brush about half of the glaze over the ham.
10. Return to the oven, uncovered, for 5 minutes, until the ham is golden brown and beginning to glaze.

11. Brush with the remaining glaze and bake for another 7 to 10 minutes, until the ham is well-browned and glazy; be careful not to let the glaze burn.
12. Serve warm.

Grilled Pork Chops with Garlic Lime Sauce

Preparation + cooking time: 30 minutes

Servings: makes 4 servings

Ingredients:
- 1/4 cup fresh lime juice
- 1 garlic clove, minced
- 1/4 teaspoon dried hot red-pepper flakes
- 1/3 cup olive oil
- 2 tablespoons chopped fresh cilantro
- 6 (1/2-inch-thick) boneless pork chops

Directions:
1. Whisk together lime juice, garlic, red-pepper flakes, and 1/4 teaspoon salt, then add oil in a slow stream, whisking well.
2. Whisk in cilantro.
3. Prepare a gas grill for direct-heat cooking over medium-high heat. Pat pork dry and season with salt and pepper.
4. Oil grill rack, then grill pork chops, covered, turning over once, until just cooked through, 5 to 6 minutes' total.
5. Serve drizzled with some vinaigrette, and with remainder on the side.

Mini Cannoli Cream Pastry Cups

Preparation + cooking time: 45 minutes

Servings: makes 48 servings

Ingredients:
- 1 container (15 oz) whole-milk ricotta cheese
- ½ cup powdered sugar
- 2 tablespoons granulated sugar
- ½ teaspoon vanilla
- 1 box Pillsbury™ refrigerated pie crusts, softened as directed on box
- 3 tablespoons turbinado sugar (raw sugar)
- 1 teaspoon ground cinnamon
- ¼ cup miniature semisweet chocolate chips
- Additional powdered sugar

Directions:
1. In large bowl, beat all filling ingredients with electric mixer on medium speed until creamy.
2. Place filling in 1-gallon resealable food-storage plastic bag; refrigerate while making cups.
3. Heat oven to 425°F. On lightly floured work surface, unroll pie crusts. Sprinkle each crust with turbinado sugar and cinnamon.
4. Lightly roll rolling pin over sugar and cinnamon to press into pastry. With 2 1/2- to 3-inch round cutter, cut out pastry rounds.
5. Lightly press each pastry round into ungreased mini muffin cup. Bake about 10 minutes or until pastry cups are golden brown.
6. Cool completely in pans, about 15 minutes. Remove from muffin cups to cooling racks.
7. Just before serving, remove filling from refrigerator.

8. Cut 1 bottom corner off bag; pipe scant tablespoon filling into cooled pastry cups.
9. Sprinkle with chocolate chips and powdered sugar. Serve immediately.
10. Store any remaining pastry cups at room temperature and filling in refrigerator

Chocolate-Peppermint Mini Cheesecakes

Preparation + cooking: 5 hours 15 minutes

Servings: makes 12 servings

Ingredients:
- 1 cup chocolate wafer cookie crumbs
- 2 Tablespoons butter, melted
- 3 pkg. (8 oz. each) PHILADELPHIA Cream Cheese, softened
- 3/4 cup sugar
- 2 teaspoons peppermint extract
- 3 eggs
- 1 package (4 oz.) BAKER'S White Chocolate, melted
- 2 oz. BAKER'S Bittersweet Chocolate
- 15 starlight mints, crushed

Directions:
1. Heat oven to 325°F.
2. Combine cookie crumbs and butter; press onto bottom of 12 (4-oz.) ovenproof glass jars. Place in shallow pan.
3. Beat cream cheese, sugar and extract in large bowl with mixer until blended. Add eggs, 1 at a time, mixing after each just until blended.
4. Stir in white chocolate; pour over crusts.
5. Bake 20 to 25 min. or until centers of cheesecakes are almost set. Cool. Refrigerate 4 hours.
6. Melt bittersweet chocolate as directed on package; drizzle over cheesecakes.
7. Sprinkle with crushed candy.

Conclusion

Weight Watchers now become as king of rapid weight lose program. Weight Watchers is aware of that it isn't just diet that will get final results. If you mix diet with workout the outcomes are a lot much more immediate and more profound.

The fact that Weight Watchers stresses the importance of physical exercise and bodily health additionally to proper diet and altering your strategy for considering in terms of food is yet a different reason for his or her widely known triumph.

Weight Watchers is just one of many diverse excess weight loss and dieting applications within the marketplace today. The fact that they've produced a name for themselves and stand out above the relaxation in numerous ways is nothing to acquire lightly. It appears that there may be a new pounds reduction system cropping up each other month or so and yet Weight Watchers continues to attain visible and sustainable final results in those that really do the job the program. Very couple of applications can make that claim for as long as Weight Watchers has been ready to.

Remember, I **am here cheering you on**, and my thoughts and my heart are with you all the way. I know you've totally got this! **I am sending you so much love and luck** on your amazing journey. Keep going, because I am here with you - all the way! Well done! And I'm sending loads of love to you.

Stay positive, always

Lots of love from **Dylan Cooper**

Printed in Great Britain
by Amazon